THE HEART DISEASE EPIDEMIC

Chapter One

This year more than 1½ million Americans will have a heart attack and half a million will die. More than 4½ million Americans have a history of coronary heart disease.[1]

This year half a million Americans will have a stroke and approximately **164,000 will die.** Americans who have had strokes and are still alive number 1,870,000.[2]

This year cardiovascular disease (disease of the heart or blood vessels) will kill almost as many Americans as *all* other causes of death combined. Approximately 43 million Americans have one or more forms of cardiovascular disease.[3]

This year experts estimate that the economic costs of cardiovascular disease will reach $64.4 billion.[4]

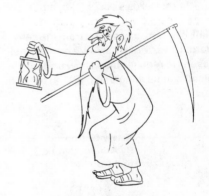

According to authorities, one in four American adults has high blood pressure, and the average American man has a one in three chance of developing some form of cardiovascular disease before age 60.

We Americans are experiencing an epidemic of cardiovascular disease. If such a steep rate of disease and death resulted from any other cause, we would call a state of national emergency. Yet, for some unfathomable reason, we stubbornly maintain our self-destructive habits *even while our diseased hearts tick our little remaining time away.*

1

RISK FACTORS IN HEART DISEASE

Factors That Cannot Be Changed	Factors That Can Be Changed or Controlled
Heredity	Cigarette smoking
	Poor nutrition
	High blood cholesterol and triglyceride levels
	High blood pressure
	Diabetes
	Obesity
	Lack of exercise
	Stress

Atherosclerosis—Key Culprit in Heart Disease

The key culprit in heart disease is a complex condition called *atherosclerosis*. Atherosclerosis is the most common form of arteriosclerosis, or "hardening of the arteries."

Atherosclerosis occurs when the linings of the arteries become thickened and hardened with accumulations of fat, cholesterol, fibrin (a clotting material), calcium, and debris from the cells. As the artery walls become thick and hard, the arteries narrow and lose their ability to contract and expand. This results in reduced blood flow through these arteries and an increased risk of a blood clot forming and blocking blood flow entirely.

Artery Narrowed By Atherosclerotic Build-Up   **Artery Blocked By Atherosclerotic Build-Up and Clot**

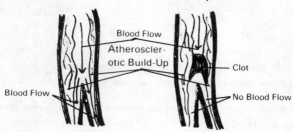

Blood Flow
Atherosclerotic Build-Up
Clot
Blood Flow
No Blood Flow

2

When a clot completely blocks an artery to the *heart*, the result is loss of blood to the heart and a *coronary thrombosis*, one form of heart attack. When a clot completely blocks an artery to the *brain*, the result is loss of blood to the brain and a *cerebral thrombosis*, one form of stroke.

Unfortunately, atherosclerosis is a silent, symptomless disease, and a person might not be aware of a problem until something dramatic happened— such as a stroke, heart failure, kidney failure, or blocked blood flow to some other part of the body (such as the legs). *Tragically, for 25 percent of heart attack victims, sudden death is the first outward sign of heart trouble.*

If all this has begun to sound pretty grim to you, I'll admit that the situation *has* been grim—at least until very recently. Happily, current research has begun to focus on this seemingly hopeless state of affairs. **A major scientific breakthrough in the prevention of atherosclerosis and heart disease is on the horizon. And heralding this breakthrough is the discovery of EPA.**

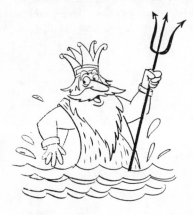

EPA—Nature's Gift to Your Heart

Recent research has turned up evidence that concentrated amounts of a nutrient found in fish oils can actually *help protect us from heart disease*. This nutrient is called *eicosapentaenoic acid,* or *EPA* for short.

EPA has been shown to reduce blood viscosity and platelet adhesiveness, so that the blood is less sticky and less prone to clot. This in turn reduces the risk of plaque formation on the walls of the arteries and clots cutting off the vital flow of blood to the heart, brain, and other parts of the body.

Before we discuss the marvels of EPA, however, we need a little background information. The starting point is an intriguing story of *Eskimos, Norwegians, Japanese, and an important discovery.*

NOTES

[1,2,3,4] American Heart Association, *Heart Facts 1984.*

THE SECRET OF THE ESKIMO

Chapter Two

For a number of years scientists and medical researchers have known that *the Eskimos of Greenland have a very low incidence of heart disease*. What they could *not* understand, however — until very recently — was *why*. Eskimos eat a large amount of whale blubber, a saturated animal fat—and saturated fat, as we know, is a significant factor in heart disease.

Lacking a better explanation, scientists hypothesized the Eskimos had some sort of inborn "genetic protection" against the effects of a high saturated fat diet. The inadequacy of this explanation became clear as members of this population group left Greenland and settled in the United States and Europe. *When these transplanted Eskimos adopted a standard Western diet, their rate of coronary heart disease increased to equal the American and European rate*. Apparently, "genetic protection" is *not* the secret of the Eskimos.

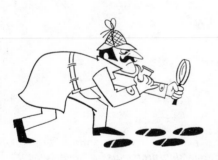

Studies Show Striking Contrasts

The first in-depth study of the Greenland Eskimos was conducted in the early 1970s by two scientists named Bang and Dyerberg.[1] They researched a district in Greenland with a population of 2,600 and found that from 1963 to 1967 there were *only three deaths from atherosclerosis*. In a subsequent study,[2] these two scientists determined that there had been *no deaths from this cause during the decade of 1968-1978*. **During this same decade, atherosclerosis was the number one cause of death among Americans!**

Intrigued by their findings, Bang and Dyerberg examined the statistics of coronary heart disease for *all* of Greenland.[3] Their study used data from 1974-1976 for males ages 45-64. This group was chosen because it contains an exceptionally high percentage of heart attack victims. The scientists compared the Greenland statistics with statistics for Americans of the same age group and sex. Their results are shown below.

Death Rates from Coronary Heart Disease[4]

Country	Coronary Heart Disease Deaths (% of all deaths)
Greenland	5.3
United States	40.4

The American population studied had nearly eight times the death rate from heart disease as the Greenland population! Furthermore, it was pointed out that the Greenland figure probably was high since it represented the total Greenland area from the "westernized" south to the native north.

What, the scientists wondered, was the Eskimo "edge"?

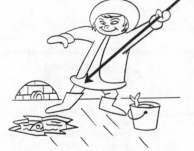

Eskimos Eat Cold Water Fish

Bang and Dyerberg diligently studied the diet of the Greenland people. After extensive surveys and research, they found *"seafood to be the back-bone of the diet."*[5] The particular *type* of seafood eaten was *cold water fish*. Much of the Eskimo diet is whale, seal, and cold water fish — obviously not the standard American fare!

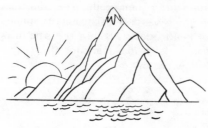

Norway: Fish Consumption Up, Heart Disease Down

Encouraged by the results of their Greenland investigation, Bang and Dyerberg looked for differences in heart disease among *other* populations that consume larger than normal amounts of cold water fish. They came across the Norwegians.[6]

The researchers found that between 1941 and 1945, during World War II, the Norwegian population in Oslo experienced a *marked decrease in heart attack deaths.* During this period, the scientists learned, Norwegian diets included a significant reduction in dairy foods and a *significant increase in cold water fish*, especially herring. Bang and Dyerberg concluded that the decrease in coronary heart disease in Oslo, Norway was due, at least in part, to this change in the Norwegian diet.[7]

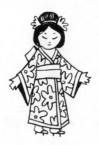

Japan: Studies Support Fish Findings

The *Japanese* rate of heart disease, though higher than the Eskimo rate, is still significantly lower than the American. The native Japanese diet, like the Eskimo, includes a *generous amount of cold water fish.*

Coastal Japanese, who eat *more* cold water fish, have a *lower* rate of heart disease than inland Japanese, who eat *less.* Both groups, however, have a *much lower* incidence of heart disease than Americans, who eat correspondingly smaller amounts of cold water fish than either group of Japanese.

Don't make the mistake of thinking (as some scientists did about the Eskimos) that the Japanese have some sort of "genetic protection" against heart disease. Studies have shown that (like the Eskimos) when Japanese settle in the United States and adopt the Standard American Diet (SAD), their rate of heart disease rises to equal the American rate.

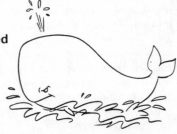

Mystery Ingredient in Fish Discovered

Scientists have come a long way from these first inspired but exploratory studies. We now know that *the vital heart-protecting element in cold water fish is its oil.* Even more exciting, we have been able to identify and isolate the primary active ingredient in this oil. This ingredient — so important to our hearts — is **EPA** — *the secret of the Eskimo.*

NOTES

[1] Bang, H.O. and J. Dyerberg. 1972. Plasma lipids and lipoproteins in Greenland west coast Eskimos. Acta. med. scand. *192*:85-94.

[2] Bang, H.O. and J. Dyerberg. 1981a. The lipid metabolism in Greenlanders. Meddr. Gronland. Man and Soc. *2*:1-18.

[3] Ibid.

[4] Ibid.

[5] Ibid.

[6] Bang, H.O. and J. Dyerberg. 1981b. Personal reflections on the incidence of ischemic heart disease in Oslo during the second world war. Acta. med. scand. *210*:245-248.

[7] Ibid.

THE MECHANICS OF HEART DISEASE

Chapter Three

Seventy-two times a minute, more than 100,000 times a day, your heart beats to keep the five or six quarts of blood in your body circulating. Over a 75-year lifespan, your heart will pump more than *18 million barrels of blood* through the vessels of your body.

The circulatory process goes like this. Your heart muscle contracts, relaxes, then contracts again, each time sending about two ounces of blood bursting into your blood vessels faster than a foot a second.

Flowing first through smooth-walled, pencil-thick, expandable arteries, the blood eventually winds its way into smaller and smaller vessels and then into millions of tiny capillaries so narrow that red blood cells can only trickle through in single file. Through the capillary walls, oxygen and nutrients from the blood are exchanged for carbon dioxide and cellular wastes. Then the trip back to the heart begins.

The blood passes back through the capillaries to the larger blood vessels and even larger veins at one-third the speed at which it began its journey. Eventually it returns to the heart and is pumped into the lungs to exchange its load of carbon dioxide for a fresh supply of oxygen. Then it returns to the heart, refreshed, to begin the cycle again.

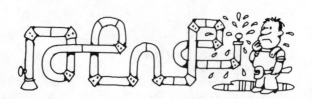

This wondrous procedure should continue for 70 years or more, even 100 years — **but there are mishaps.** *A breakdown occurs in the system...the rhythm is broken, and the heartbeat is delayed or even halted.* What goes wrong? What causes such a breakdown, and does it have to occur?

Plaque: One Kink
In the Circulatory System

Often what happens to cause the breakdown is that the circulatory system becomes clogged or choked through *atherosclerosis*. Atherosclerosis occurs when yellowish, fatty deposits — called *plaque* — accumulate in and on the inner walls of the arteries. Plaque is made up of fat, cholesterol, fibrin (a clotting substance), calcium, and cellular debris. **As a result of plaque accumulation, the arteries become thick and hard and blood cannot flow easily through them.**

Plaque can build up in an artery until it cuts off the flow of blood entirely. Plaque can also narrow arteries so much that a *blood clot* wedged between the walls of an artery can cut off blood flow through that artery.

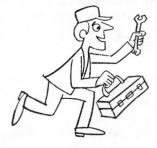

Blood Clots: A Second Kink
In the System

The major way the circulatory system can suffer a breakdown is through *blood clotting*. A clot that forms in a blood vessel can block the flow of blood just as surely as though you pinched the vessel shut. Because blood clots can be so dangerous, we will discuss them in greater detail a little later. For now, though, this is integral: **Blood must be kept flowing. Anything that cuts off blood flow is dangerous and potentially deadly.**

When parts of the body are cut off from their blood supply they begin to die. Brain tissue can survive only about four minutes without blood. Heart tissue can hold out only 20 to 40 minutes. No cells can last longer than one hour without their needed blood supply.

The results of cut-off blood flow are known by a variety of names: *myocardial infarction* (damage to the heart muscle that produces the classic *coronary* or heart attack), *stroke* (damage to or destruction of a part of the brain), *angina pectoris* (chest pains that can lead to serious and sometimes fatal *tachycardia* or *fibrillation*), and more.

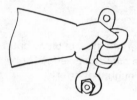

The Nuts and Bolts of Heart Disease: Some Definitions

It would make sense, then, for us to do all we can to prevent the accumulation of plaque and the formation of blood clots in our arteries.

To understand the mechanics of blood clot formation requires our familiarity with some important terms. Following are some helpful definitions. Please refer to these as necessary.

Vocabulary

Eicosapentaenoic Acid - An essential fatty acid found mainly in cold water fish.

Blood Platelets - Tiny particles in the blood responsible for blood clotting.

Omega-3 Fatty Acids - For our purposes, a group of fatty acids found mainly in cold water fish. EPA is an omega-3 fatty acid.

Omega-6 Fatty Acids - A group of fatty acids found predominantly in the Standard American Diet (SAD).

Vasoconstrictor - A substance which constricts blood vessels or causes them to decrease in diameter.

Thromboxane A - A chemical in blood platelets that begins the blood clot. It is also a vasoconstrictor. There are two types of thromboxane. Thromboxane A_2 is *very prone* to form clots and is a *strong* vasoconstrictor. Thromboxane A_3 is *not so prone* to form clots and is *less* of a vasoconstrictor.

10

Cholesterol - The fatty substance in our systems that can cause plaque (fatty build-up in the arteries). It is good to have a low total cholesterol level, but not all cholesterol is created equal. There are two major types of cholesterol.

LDL and HDL Cholesterol - LDL cholesterol takes cholesterol from the liver to the tissues. HDL cholesterol takes cholesterol from the tissues to the liver for destruction. To make it easy, LDL are the "bad guys" and HDL are the "good guys."

CHOLESTEROL

TWO TYPES - LDL & HDL

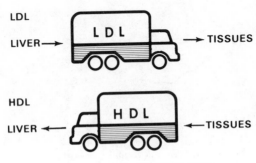

LOW SERUM CHOLESTEROL IS GOOD

BUT

THE HIGHER THE HDL RELATIVE TO THE LDL, THE LOWER THE RISK OF A HEART ATTACK AT ANY AGE.

Preventing Plaque Accumulation

An important element in avoiding cardiovascular disease, as we've seen, is preventing the accumulation of plaque. While we can't *guarantee* its elimination, we can take certain *precautions* against its development. One precaution is to reduce our total fat and cholesterol intake and to substitute unsaturated fats for saturated fats in our diet. In the next chapter we'll discuss a special kind of unsaturated fat that can work best in our systems.

A second precaution against plaque is to intensify our exercise, and a third is to increase our dietary fiber.

A fourth step is to supplement our diets with two important nutrients, EPA and lecithin. We'll talk more about the special significance of these two nutrients later in this book.

The Blood Clotting Process

The major element in avoiding cardiovascular disease is preventing the formation of dangerous blood clots. Let's take a look now at the blood clotting process.

Blood clotting is controlled by tiny particles in the blood called *platelets*. These tiny particles (about one billion per teaspoon of blood) are called platelets because they resemble *plates,* and like plates, they are fragile. Their primary purpose is to put a stop to bleeding, and to do so they initially clump together to form plugs, called *pre-clots* or *aggregates.*

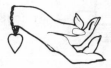

When you cut your finger, you injure blood vessels in the finger, under the skin, causing blood to leak out. Your fragile platelets respond to this injury by cracking or breaking and releasing a substance called *thromboxane.* Thromboxane causes the platelets to become sticky and clump together in masses of pre-clots or aggregates. These masses of platelets race to the leak in the blood vessel and plug it up, much like a "stop leak" compound in a radiator.

If the cut to your finger is small, the platelets will only crack — not break —and release small amounts of thromboxane. If the cut is large, the platelets will break and release large amounts of thromboxane. In general, the more thromboxane released, the more the platelets will clump together, and the more "sophisticated" the clot will become. (I say *in general* because actually there are *two kinds of thromboxane,* and each will react differently. The importance of this difference will become clear a little later.)

Thromboxane also causes the injured blood vessel to become constricted, or narrowed, thus helping to stop the loss of blood in another manner.

PLATELET
AGGREGATION

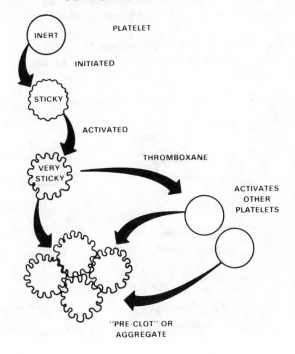

Dangers of Overreactive Platelets

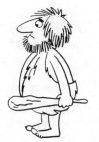

Thousands of years ago our fragile platelets served us well. After an encounter with a saber-toothed tiger, we *needed* a rapid blood-clotting mechanism to prevent our bleeding to death. Now, however, **our trigger-happy platelets can often be more harmful than helpful**. In fact, they can sometimes be downright *deadly*.

Suppose you develop a blood clot *inside* a blood vessel. The clot could restrict or block entirely the flow of blood through that vessel, and the result could be serious damage to a part of the body normally supplied by that vessel and cut off by the clot from its needed blood supply.

Picture a blood clot in a coronary artery coupled with an extreme narrowing of the artery caused by the release of thromboxane. The result could be a massive coronary — heart attack — and possible death.

Here are four ways overreactive blood platelets can be dangerous to our heart and circulatory system. The following diagram illustrates each of these four instances.

PLATELET PROBLEMS

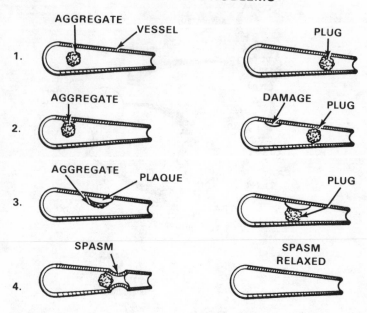

1. Overreactive platelets can form an *aggregate* (a clump) that can lodge in the naturally narrow part of a blood vessel — *and block the flow of blood.*

2. Very slight damage to a blood vessel can cause an aggregate to form, and the aggregate can then break off from the vessel wall — *and block the flow of blood.*

3. An aggregate can form on plaque, grow in size — *and block the flow of blood.*

4. An aggregate can get squeezed between the walls of an artery due to a spasm in the artery caused by the release of thromboxane — *and block the flow of blood.*

The Answer to Overreactive Platelets

It seems apparent that the answer to our problem of overreactive platelets is somehow to make them *less fragile* (or *sensitive*.) **The less fragile (or sensitive) our platelets are, the less chance they'll be activated to break or crack and form unwanted blood clots.**

A fine china plate is very fragile and breaks or cracks easily. Other dinner plates designed for heavier use are less fragile and more difficult to damage. *Our bodies can produce fragile platelets or less fragile platelets.*

What can we do to make our platelets less fragile? The answer lies in thromboxane, and the secret is EPA.

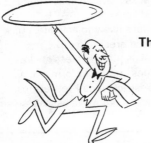

Thromboxane Makes the Difference

You'll recall from our discussion of blood clotting that *thromboxane* is a substance released by the platelets when they crack or break. There are two kinds of thromboxane that are of particular concern to us here. One kind is *thromboxane A_2. Thromboxane A_2 inside a platelet makes it more fragile or sensitive and more likely to crack or break.* When thromboxane A_2 is released upon a platelet's cracking or breaking, *it makes the platelets stickier and more prone to aggregate, or form blood clots.*

The second kind of thromboxane is *thromboxane A_3. Thromboxane A_3 inside a platelet makes it less fragile or sensitive and less likely to crack or break.* When a sturdy platelet still cracks or breaks, the thromboxane A_3 it releases will *not cause platelets to stick together as much as thromboxane A_2 will.* The less sticky the platelets become, the less risk they'll aggregate and form a dangerous blood clot.

Thus we've seen two ways the kind of thromboxane in our platelets can be especially important. There's a third way, as well.

Thromboxane A₂ is a potent vasoconstrictor. It causes the blood vessels to become constricted (narrowed), so less blood can flow through them. *Thromboxane A₃ is a less potent vasoconstrictor.* When released from the platelets, thromboxane A_3 is less likely to narrow blood vessels and restrict blood flow. Since our goal is to keep the blood flowing smoothly through our blood vessels, we seldom would want the vessels to become constricted.

For simplicity, let's refer to thromboxane A_2 as *unwanted thromboxane* and thromboxane A_3 as *wanted thromboxane.* Now we'll quickly review the differences between unwanted thromboxane and wanted thromboxane.

Unwanted Thromboxane (A_2)	Wanted Thromboxane (A_3)
Makes platelets more fragile and sensitive (more likely to activate, crack and break)	Makes platelets less fragile and sensitive (less likely to activate, crack and break)
Makes platelets stickier (more prone to form clots)	Makes platelets less sticky (less prone to form clots)
Constricts blood vessels more (makes vessels smaller)	Constricts blood vessels less (does not make vessels so small)

Obviously our goal is to get more wanted thromboxane A₃ and less unwanted thromboxane A₂ into our platelets. Fortunately, there's a simple, effective way to do this. It has to do with EPA and the kind of fat we eat.

Thromboxane and Fatty Acids

For our purposes, we can limit our discussion of fats to two kinds of fatty acids — *omega-6 and omega-3.* Omega-6 fatty acids are commonly found in the Standard American Diet. Omega-3 fatty acids, preponderant in cold water fish oils, are less frequently found in the American diet.

Omega-6 fatty acids when processed by the body produce unwanted thromboxane A_2. Omega-3 fatty acids when processed by the body produce wanted thromboxane A_3. Therefore, to increase the wanted thromboxane in our platelets, we need to ingest more omega-3 fatty acids. We can do this by eating considerably more cold water fish, or we can use a product derived from the oil of cold water fish. This product is called *eicosapentaenoic acid,* or *EPA.*

ALL PUT TOGETHER

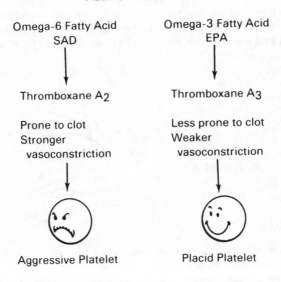

Omega-6 Fatty Acid SAD	Omega-3 Fatty Acid EPA
↓	↓
Thromboxane A_2	Thromboxane A_3
Prone to clot Stronger vasoconstriction	Less prone to clot Weaker vasoconstriction
Aggressive Platelet	Placid Platelet

EPA

Through the manufacture of wanted thromboxane A_3, EPA can make our platelets less fragile and less prone to aggregate and form harmful blood clots within the arteries. It also can reduce the tendency of our blood vessels to narrow and restrict vital blood flow.

For these reasons *alone,* we would certainly want to insure an adequate intake of EPA. Yet EPA can work wonders for our heart and blood vessels in *other* ways as well.

Now turn with me to Chapter Four, where we will discuss *additional* benefits that can come from this amazing nutrient.

EPA — NUTRITION BREAKTHROUGH
IN HEART DISEASE

Chapter Four

In the last chapter we saw how EPA can help prevent deadly blood clots from forming and blocking vital blood flow. In this chapter we'll learn even more about EPA and the additional ways it can protect our heart and circulatory system.

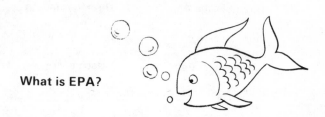

What is EPA?

EPA is short for *eicosapentaenoic acid,* a polyunsaturated omega-3 fatty acid that comes primarily from cold water fish. Omega-3 fatty acids, you'll recall, produce *wanted thromboxane A_3* in our blood platelets. Omega-6 fatty acids, predominant in our Standard American Diet (SAD), produce *unwanted thromboxane A_2.* Let's quickly review that process.

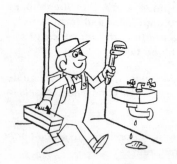

EPA Inhibits Harmful Blood Clotting

As an omega-3 fatty acid, EPA in the body produces thromboxane A_3. Thromboxane A_3 — *wanted thromboxane* — produces platelets that are sturdier and less prone to clot. Thromboxane A_3 also is a less potent vasoconstrictor (artery-narrower) than thromboxane A_2, so blood can flow more easily through the arteries.

The following chart summarizes the effects of EPA on the blood clotting process.

COMPARISON OF OMEGA-3 AND OMEGA-6 FATTY ACIDS ON BLOOD CLOTTING PROCESS

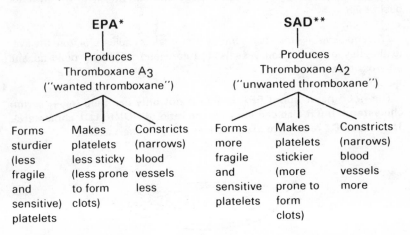

Dietary Omega-3 Fatty Acids   **Dietary Omega-6 Fatty Acids**

EPA*   SAD**

Produces   Produces
Thromboxane A$_3$ Thromboxane A$_2$
("wanted thromboxane")   ("unwanted thromboxane")

Forms	Makes	Constricts	Forms	Makes	Constricts
sturdier	platelets	(narrows)	more	platelets	(narrows)
(less	less sticky	blood	fragile	stickier	blood
fragile	(less prone	vessels	and	(more	vessels
and	to form	less	sensitive	prone to	more
sensitive)	clots)		platelets	form	
platelets				clots)	

---

*Eicosapentaenoic acid
**Standard American Diet

When we realize that 90 percent of the time, a heart attack does not occur until a blood clot forms and blocks a blood vessel, the importance of EPA becomes apparent. In general, no clot, no heart attack.

Here is a quotation from the Tufts University *Diet and Nutrition News Letter,* August 1984: "A number of studies show that eating large amounts of omega three fatty acids can decrease the tendency of blood platelet cells, involved with the clotting, to stick or clump together. This decreases the likelihood of forming clots that can block blood flow to the heart, resulting in a heart attack. The omega three fatty acids have also been shown to decrease blood levels of the fatty triglycerides and cholesterol, both associated with cardiovascular disease." [1]

EPA Reduces Serum Cholesterol, Improves Cholesterol Balance

Cholesterol is the fatty substance in our systems that can cause plaque and subsequent atherosclerosis. We want to have a low serum (blood) cholesterol level, but we also want to achieve a healthy ratio between the two major kinds of cholesterol, HDL and LDL.

HDL cholesterol is the "good" cholesterol. It helps rid the body of unwanted cholesterol by taking it from the tissues and carrying it to the liver for destruction.

LDL cholesterol is the "bad" cholesterol. It takes cholesterol from the liver to the tissues and blood vessels and can lead to plaque build-up and atherosclerosis.

The good news about EPA is that it not only can help lower serum cholesterol, but it also can improve the ratio of HDL to LDL cholesterol. The more HDL relative to LDL, the less risk of a heart attack.

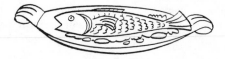

In an article in the prestigious medical journal *Lancet,* June 11, 1983, the British scientist, Dr. Reginald Saynor, reported research he had conducted since 1980 on fish oil concentrates (a prime source of EPA). At the time of the article Saynor had studied 150 people who had been supplementing their diets for as long as three years with fish oil concentrates.

"The participants," he wrote, "include patients who have had myocardial infarction [heart attack], patients with angina, and symptomless volunteers. Some patients had had coronary artery bypass surgery or coronary dilatation.

"After the subjects had been taking the oil two years...The total serum cholesterol was significantly lower...and the HDL cholesterol was significantly higher." [2]

Another important study, conducted at the University of Oregon Health Sciences Center in Portland, demonstrated similar results. After a ten-day diet of salmon (rich in omega-3 fatty acids), presumably healthy volunteers showed a *17 percent drop in plasma cholesterol levels*. Patients with elevated cholesterol experienced a drop of *20 percent or more.* [3]

Just by adding omega-3 fatty acids to our diets we apparently can effect some dramatic shifts in our cholesterol levels!

EPA Decreases Triglyceride Levels

A high serum triglyceride level has long been associated with cardiovascular disease. Numerous methods have been tried to reduce triglycerides, but all have had poor results. The usual advice is to lose weight and increase exercise. What effect has EPA had in this area?

In the journal *Metabolism,* February 1983, Dr. William Harris and his colleagues reported on the effects of omega-3 fatty acids on triglycerides. (Remember that EPA is an omega-3 fatty acid.) The researchers checked their subjects' triglyceride levels throughout the study, and *what they found was tremendously exciting.* Those subjects whose diets were high in omega-3 fatty acids experienced a drop in triglyceride levels heretofore thought *nearly impossible.* **Their triglycerides were reduced by an astounding 33 percent below the control group.** [4]

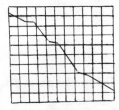

"No other polyunsaturated oils have been able to get triglyceride levels to drop in this way," said Dr. Harris. "So the impact of the fish-oil diet is really significant. For a person with high triglyceride levels, a 33 percent reduction would be an important change toward better cardiovascular health."

The study we referred to earlier, at the University of Oregon, also reported on triglyceride levels. After their 10-day diet of salmon, the healthy volunteers showed a triglyceride drop of as much as *40 percent.* Patients with mildly elevated triglyceride levels saw their triglyceride levels fall by as much as *67 percent! All this after only ten days!*

Considering that until this time we have had such poor results from our attempts to lower triglycerides, **these findings are immensely impressive. Increasing omega-3 fatty acids in our diets could have tremendous positive impact on our triglyceride levels.**

EPA Can Lower High Blood Pressure

Additional studies indicate that EPA, an omega-3 fatty acid, may prove **even more valuable** in cardiovascular health. **Omega-3 fatty acids also have been shown to reduce high blood pressure.** As you know, high blood pressure is associated with a number of cardiovascular problems, including heart attacks and strokes.

How does EPA lower high blood pressure? We don't have the whole answer yet, but it apparently works in at least four ways.
- It makes the blood less viscous (less thick) so it can flow easier and with less resistance through the blood vessels.
- Through the production of wanted thromboxane A_3 it has less of a narrowing effect on blood vessels.
- Through the production of thromboxane A_3 it allows for better control of norepinephrine, a potent vasoconstrictor.
- It lowers the kidney's output of renin, another vasoconstrictor.

An article in *Circulation,* an official journal of the American Heart Association, cited the beneficial effects of omega-3 fatty acids on high blood pressure. In the study reported, subjects maintained a standard American diet but took omega-3 fatty acid supplements. Their overall blood pressure dropped, with their systolic blood pressure dropping an average of nearly *10 points.* [5]
When you recall that one in four American adults has high blood pressure, you can't help but realize the significance of EPA's blood pressure lowering function.

What Do the Experts Think?

Now that we've seen all the ways EPA can benefit our heart and blood vessels, it looks like quite an impressive nutrient. But what do the experts think?

Consider this statement by Donald O. Rudin, M.D., former director of the molecular biology department at Eastern Pennsylvania Psychiatric Institute in Philadelphia.

"After years of research," said Dr. Rudin, "we now know that omega-3 fatty acids are absolutely required by the body. They're not optional nutrients. Yet most of the population is deficient in them. The consumption of cholesterol and fat is way up at a time when omega-3 consumption is way down. We obviously need these fatty acids more than ever. They're the last major nutrient family to be recognized. In more ways than one, they're our nutritional missing link."

This is a strong statement, but after reading reams of research on omega-3 fatty acids and their potential benefits, I could not agree more with Dr. Rudin.

SUMMARY OF POTENTIAL BENEFITS OF EPA ON CARDIOVASCULAR HEALTH

1. Reduces serum cholesterol levels
2. Reduces serum triglyceride levels
3. Lowers blood pressure if high
4. Decreases (the bad) LDL cholesterol
5. Increases (the good) HDL cholesterol
6. Reduces the risk of harmful blood clot formation
7. Reduces blood viscosity and platelet adhesiveness
8. Reduces the risk of cardiovascular disease

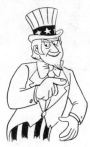

American Diets Deficient in EPA

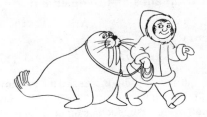

With all these potential health benefits, we certainly want to get a good amount of EPA in our diets. *Yet Americans — and most people in the Western world — are not getting even close to adequate amounts of EPA.* Is *any* population group getting enough of this important nutrient? Yes, you'll recall there is one group, in particular, that gets an abundance of EPA in its food. This group is the *Eskimos of Greenland.*

How to Increase EPA Intake

Does this mean we have to eat like the Eskimos to get a good amount of EPA in our diet? No, not necessarily.

We *can* choose, as some scientists have done, to adopt an Eskimo diet. (For the life of me, though, I can't figure out where to buy whale blubber!) Eating more mackerel, sardines, salmon, cod, or other fatty fish *will* increase our intake of EPA. However, getting optimum quantities of EPA from our food could mean eating as much as *a pound of salmon or two cans of mackerel each day!* Will a "Big Mackerel" become a new hit at the fast food chains? Somehow, I doubt it.

I am often asked whether we must change our dietary lifestyle to get the benefits of EPA. Fortunately, the answer is *no*. Just a little EPA added to our Standard American Diet can result in many beneficial changes.

We *could* choose to increase our intake of cod liver oil; it contains EPA. But cod liver oil has three strikes against it. One strike is that most people *can't stand the taste*. The second, even more important, strike is that cod liver oil contains significant amounts of vitamins A and D, and *these vitamins can be toxic in large amounts*. The third strike against cod liver oil is that it contains some 20- and 22-carbon compounds that can actually *cause heart problems*.

Our third choice, and the one that makes the most sense to me, is to use an EPA supplement in capsule form.

Thank goodness for
EPA supplements

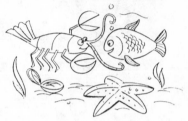

Advantages of a Supplement

Although I *have* increased the amount of cold water fish in my diet, there's still a *limit* to how much fish I'll eat. Also, there are times I'm unable to eat cold water fish, such as on an airplane or just before a "face to face" social event. ("Sardine breath" could ruin my social life!)

Taking a supplement insures my getting an optimal amount of EPA each day and gives me the flexibility and convenience I need in 20th century America.

A Good EPA Supplement

Generally, a good EPA supplement will contain a high concentration of EPA and a percentage of another omega-3 fatty acid we have not mentioned, *docosahexaenoic acid (DHA)*. This particular fatty acid makes EPA work more effectively.

I'm convinced that EPA is Nature's gift to our hearts. I encourage you to take what Nature wants you to have — *EPA, a special nutrient for a healthy heart.*

NOTES

[1] Tufts University *Diet and Nutrition News Letter,* August 1984.
[2] *Lancet,* June 11, 1983.
[3] *Journal of the American Medical Association,* Feb. 12, 1982.
[4] *Metabolism,* February 1983.
[5] *Circulation,* Volume 67, No. 3, March 1983.

THE LECITHIN ADVANTAGE

Chapter Five

In this chapter I want to call your attention to another nutrient that, together with EPA, *can really work wonders* for your heart and circulatory system. This nutrient is *lecithin*.

Lecithin benefits the heart and circulatory system in ways similar to EPA, but **through entirely different biological and physiological processes. Because it works in different ways from EPA, lecithin can be especially useful when taken along with EPA.**

What is Lecithin?

Lecithin (pronounced *less-ih-thin*) is a nutrient found naturally in plant and animal tissues and produced commercially from soybeans, corn oil, or egg yolks. It is an excellent source of *linoleic acid,* an *essential* fatty acid required by the body to metabolize cholesterol, triglycerides, and other lipids. Because our bodies cannot manufacture linoleic acid, we must get it from the food we eat. **Lecithin is a supreme source of linoleic acid.**

Even beyond supplying us with this essential fatty acid, however, lecithin can do wonderful things for our heart and blood vessels. That's why it's so important when taken along with EPA. Let's see what lecithin can do for us.

Lecithin's Role in Cardiovascular Health

Lecithin can help in the control of triglyceride levels, reduce total serum cholesterol, and lower the LDL type while raising the HDL type. As you'll recall, high triglyceride and serum cholesterol levels are significant risk factors in cardiovascular disease. You'll also recall that we want to *increase* the ratio of HDL to LDL cholesterol in our blood. LDL cholesterol is the "bad" cholesterol that can accumulate in the arteries and lead to atherosclerosis and heart disease. HDL cholesterol is the "good" cholesterol that can actually pick up the LDL cholesterol from the tissues and arteries and take it to the liver for destruction.

If we can decrease LDL cholesterol while we increase HDL cholesterol in our blood, we'll have a far better chance of avoiding cardiovascular disease. This is precisely what lecithin can do for us.

Studies Show Lecithin's Effectiveness

Numerous studies throughout the world have demonstrated lecithin's beneficial effects. Especially important are the studies showing lecithin's effectiveness in changing the proportion of HDL to LDL cholesterol. Let's quickly look at just a few of these studies.

Sweden, 1974 — Five 50-year-old men took 1.7 grams of lecithin per day for nine weeks and abstained from alcohol. Their HDL levels went up an average of 30 percent. [1]

Australia, 1977 — Three healthy volunteers and seven patients with high cholesterol levels took lecithin for eight weeks to 11 months. One of the healthy volunteers and three of the patients evidenced a significant drop in cholesterol. This drop was almost completely accounted for by a reduction in LDL levels. [2]

Seattle, Washington, 1977 — Twelve volunteers with normal cholesterol levels took lecithin for five successive three-week periods. Their HDL levels increased by an average of 3.6 percent and their LDL levels decreased by 7 percent. [3]

Lecithin not only can reduce total serum cholesterol, but also — and even more importantly — lecithin can improve the balance between HDL and LDL in favor of the good HDL type of cholesterol.

How Lecithin Works

We mentioned already that lecithin works in **different ways from EPA.** This is the reason *both* nutrients are especially important to our cardiovascular health and the reason they work *together* so well.

Scientists postulate several mechanisms may account for lecithin's effectiveness. Some researchers believe the key is lecithin's large proportion of *linoleic acid.* As a polyunsaturated fatty acid, linoleic acid can aid in lowering elevated cholesterol levels.

Other researchers believe lecithin's benefits may derive from its supply of *choline.* Still others think both substances may be at work.

Lecithin apparently plays a twofold role in cholesterol transport. First, before cholesterol has a chance to accumulate in the arteries, lecithin stimulates its transport to the liver. Second, after cholesterol has *already* accumulated in the arteries, lecithin spurs the production of an enzyme called *LCAT* (lecithin acetyl transferase) that dissolves the accumulated cholesterol and again stimulates its transport to the liver. In both cases, once cholesterol is taken to the liver, it is used *healthfully* for bile production.

These two beneficial mechanisms work entirely differently from, and in addition to, those of EPA.

Additional Benefits

Besides its association with cardiovascular health, lecithin is involved in numerous additional bodily processes. Here are a few:

- Lecithin forms part of the myelin sheath around some nerves that speeds nerve transmission.
- It helps prevent fatty infiltration of the liver.
- It aids in the absorption and transportation of the fat-soluble vitamins A, D, E, and K.
- It helps prevent gallstones.
- In some cases it can aid short-term memory.

Sources of Lecithin

Lecithin can be produced commercially from soybeans, corn oil, or egg yolks. The best source, I find, is *soybeans.*

Studies have shown that the kind of lecithin we get from egg yolks — saturated lecithin — is not nearly as effective as unsaturated lecithin in cleaning accumulated cholesterol from the arteries.[4] Thus, I rule out egg yolks as a good source of lecithin.

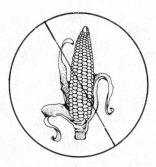 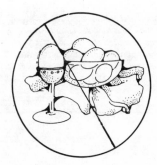

Other studies have shown that lecithin from corn oil produces little change in HDL cholesterol levels.[5] Thus, I rule out corn oil as a good source of lecithin.

That leaves soybeans. Lecithin from soybeans *does* increase HDL cholesterol, *does* decrease LDL cholesterol, and *does* help clean accumulated cholesterol from the arteries. To my mind, **soybean lecithin clearly is the lecithin of choice.**

Should You Supplement?

Lecithin seems to work best in those who need it most — persons who already have a relatively high cholesterol count. For these people, lecithin — taken with EPA — could have a very beneficial effect on cholesterol levels. Obviously, though, lecithin will affect different persons differently. For some it will have a dramatic effect; for others the effect will be less spectacular.

Should *you* take a lecithin supplement? *I do.* Personally, I prefer the preventative route to the treatment route: I'd rather take measures against high cholesterol and heart disease before it develops. **I take soybean lecithin along with EPA because I believe they work together most effectively to protect my heart and circulatory system.** *And I believe in nutrition protection.*

As for the cost of these and other nutrition supplements, I have a simple cost effective gauge. It's a question I ask myself to keep the issue of cost in perspective. **Which do you think costs more — paying a few cents each day for nutrition protection, or paying several thousand dollars one day for a coronary bypass operation?**

Think about it.

NOTES

[1] *Nutrition and Metabolism,* Vol. 17, No. 6.
[2] *Australian and New Zealand Journal of Medicine,* June 1977.
[3] *Clinical Research,* Vol. 25, No. 2, 1977.
[4] Research performed by Charles E. Butterworth, Jr., M.D., and Carlos Krumdieck, M.D., University of Alabama School of Medicine.
[5] *Atherosclerosis,* 1981.